Sinus Problems STOP!

The Complete Guide on Sinus Infection, Sinusitis Symptoms, Sinusitis Treatment, & Secrets to Natural Sinus Relief without Harsh Drugs

Susan E. Asmus

Copyright© 2014 by Susan E. Asmus

Sinus Problems STOP!

Copyright© 2014 Susan E. Asmus

All Rights Reserved.
Warning: The unauthorized reproduction or distribution of this copyrighted work is illegal. No part of this book may be scanned, uploaded or distributed via internet or other means, electronic or print without the author's permission. Criminal copyright infringement without monetary gain is investigated by the FBI and is punishable by up to 5 years in federal prison and a fine of $250,000. (http://www.fbi.gov/ipr/). Please purchase only authorized electronic or print editions and do not participate in or encourage the electronic piracy of copyrighted material.

Publisher: Enlightened Publishing

ISBN-13: 978-1500150389

ISBN-10: 150015038X

Disclaimer

The Publisher has strived to be as accurate and complete as possible in the creation of this book. While all attempts have been made to verify information provided in this publication, the Publisher assumes no responsibility for errors, omissions, or contrary interpretation of the subject matter herein. Any perceived slights of specific persons, peoples, or organizations are unintentional.

This book is not intended for use as a source of legal, business, accounting or financial advice. All readers are advised to seek services of competent professionals in the legal, business, accounting, and finance fields.

The information in this book is not intended or implied to be a substitute for professional medical advice, diagnosis or treatment. All content contained in this book is for general information purposes only. Always consult your healthcare provider before carrying on any health program.

Table of Contents

Chapter 1: Sinus Problems – Symptoms & Causes... 3

    Symptoms and Causes of Sinusitis.............. 3

    Risk Factors 9

    Complications... 11

    Conventional Medical Treatments 13

Chapter 2: Sinusitis Relief with Diet 19

    Food Allergy and Diet.................................. 19

    Food Allergy and Sinus Problems............. 20

    Food Intolerance and Sinus Problems....... 22

    Ingredients in Food to Avoid 22

Chapter 3: Sinusitis Relief with Nutritional Supplements 27

Chapter 4: Sinusitis Relief with Herbal Remedies 33

Chapter 5: Sinusitis Relief with Home Remedies 39

Neti Pot 39

Clean the Air 41

Steam 42

Avoid Perfumes and Scented Hair Oils 43

Compresses 44

Horseradish 45

Chapter 6: Sinusitis Relief with Alternative Therapies 47

Acupuncture 47

Acupressure 50

Reflexology 51

Massage 54

Ayurvedic Medicine 57

Other Homeopathic Cures for Sinusitis 60

Summary 65

Chapter 1: Sinus Problems – Symptoms & Causes

Symptoms and Causes of Sinusitis

To understand what sinusitis is, one must understand what sinuses are in the first place. In essence, there are hollow spaces behind the face; these are sinuses. To be more specific, directly behind the nose is the nasal cavity, and on either side of it are two large sinuses. Two more are located above and behind the inner part of the eyebrows and there is a small row of sinuses along the ridge of the nose.

In short, sinuses are natural air filters; their job is to protect our respiratory pathways from the airborne pathogens which are present in the air on any given day. They filter out bacteria, dust, viruses, and pollen and protect our lungs in that manner. When the sinuses become inflamed and congested, they are no longer able to effectively do their job.

Anything can cause swelling in the nose and therefore, there are many possibilities as to what can cause an obstruction in the nasal passages and sinuses. Possibilities include allergens, exposure to a chemical, or a cold. Mucus and air becomes trapped and therefore, this can cause pain in both the nasal passages and the sinus cavities.

Sinusitis pain occurs when the pressure of the thickened mucus and trapped air presses against the swollen mucous membrane and the bony ridge of the sinus behind it. Mucus gets thicker as it becomes trapped because it loses its water content, and therefore, it becomes more challenging to allow the mucus to escape effectively between the swelling and blocked nasal passages.

The bottom line is, sinus issues can be a symptom of something more invasive than a cold. Sinusitis means that the sinuses have become inflamed. There are three main causes of sinusitis; bacterial infections, viral infections or non-infectious causes. Sinusitis affects the cavities behind your nasal passages and can be either chronic or acute.

Acute sinusitis generally lasts no longer than four weeks and can be caused by the common cold, pre-existing health conditions or allergies and allergic conditions. If the cold leads to a bacterial infection, then a diagnosis of acute sinusitis can be made. Allergies and allergic conditions can cause the mucous membranes to become inflamed and therefore mucous membranes can then cause an obstruction in the nasal passages. Pre-existing health conditions such as primary immune deficiency disease or HIV, as well as cystic fibrosis, can cause greater than normal mucous secretions and that, in turn, can lead to sinusitis. Sometimes, the mucus that drains from the sinuses may also drain to the back of the throat, resulting in a condition called postnasal drip.

Chronic sinusitis may last eight to twelve weeks or even longer. It may be caused by pre-existing health conditions, as acute sinusitis is, recurrent cases of acute sinusitis, or asthma and allergies. Constant exposure to airborne allergens can cause persistent inflammation of the nasal passages and sinus cavities, which then, in turn, can create significant issues with inflammation or swelling in the nose – a sure sign of sinusitis. For a diagnosis of chronic sinusitis, at least two of the following symptoms must be present:

- Low grade fever;

- Drainage of thick, yellowish or greenish mucous from the nose or down the back of the throat;

- Nasal obstruction or congestion;

- Pain, sensitivity, or swelling around the nose, eyes or forehead;

- Reduced sense of smell and/or taste.

These, however, are not the only symptoms. Ear pain may be another common symptom; generally, as the nose becomes congested, the Eustachian tubes in the ears can also swell and become irritated from the infection. A cough, due to the mucus dripping into the back of the throat, can also be present and prevent sleep at night due to worsening symptoms. Fatigue and irritability will doubtless result, though this would be more of a symptom from the lack of sleep than anything else. Halitosis (bad breath) may also occur, because the person may be breathing through their mouth in order to feel he or she is getting enough oxygen. Finally, nausea due to a combination of these factors may result.

It should be kept in mind, however, that a doctor still needs to be seen if the following conditions don't appear to be improving or appear to be worsening:

- Pain or swelling around the eyes;

- Increased irritability;

- Swollen forehead;

- Shortness of breath;

- Severe headache;

- Double vision; and

- Confusion.

While the symptoms of sinusitis are uncomfortable, the underlying causes of the condition may be equally uncomfortable and quite serious. Nasal polyps or tumors may be a cause behind the sinusitis. A polyp is a grapelike tissue growth which can cause a fair bit of obstruction and block the flow of oxygen or mucous. Allergic responses can be triggered as a result of a fungal sinus infection.

In fact, research from the Mayo Clinic, one of the premier medical facilities in the United

States, has indicated that fungus is the most common cause to most sinusitis cases. Some 37 million people every year deal with sinusitis, and the study, conducted by the Mayo Clinic, says that some ten percent of the population of sinusitis sufferers have sinusitis which has developed from fungal infections.

In fact, of 210 patients studied, nearly 96 percent of patients dealing with sinusitis had fungus of some sort in their nasal passages or sinus cavities, which is remarkable, given it was never believed that fungal infections had played much of a role in sinusitis. It was always suspected that bacteria were the chief cause behind most sinus infections and therefore, sinusitis. Generally speaking, antibiotics are ineffective when the sinusitis has an underlying cause of a fungal infection. Antibiotics target bacteria, not fungi; as a result, sinusitis symptoms remain and may worsen, as they are not being treated adequately. Worse still, the underlying cause of the problem remains without discovery.

Thousands of fungi are found worldwide, so the methods of being able to narrow down which fungus in particular is responsible for the sinusitis becomes challenging at best, impossible at the worst. Also, with no real method to treat a nasal fungal infection, the treatment for the sinusitis is further complicated. Without treatment of the underlying causes, the sinusitis can grow worse and create more pain.

A deviated septum – the wall of tissue which splits the nostrils – can restrict or block sinus passages. As can be expected, any sort of trauma to the face which may block sinus passages can also be a contributing factor to the development of sinusitis, as the nose or nostrils may become blocked or damaged as a result of the trauma.

Risk Factors

Of course, with every infection, illness, or disease comes a variety of risk factors which can significantly impact your chances of having a problem. One in seven Americans is diagnosed with sinusitis yearly. Therefore, the infection affects roughly 44 million Americans per year.

In addition to the above symptoms, having asthma is a consideration, to an extent, of a person's probability of having chronic sinusitis. In fact, one out of five people with chronic sinusitis have asthma. A medical condition, such as cystic fibrosis or Chronic Obstructive Pulmonary Disorder (COPD) can affect your chances of having chronic sinusitis.

Regular exposure to a wide range of pollutants can affect your sensitivity to contracting sinusitis. In fact, aspirin sensitivity which can cause respiratory issues can also give you a higher-than-normal chance of developing the infection. Gastroesophogeal reflux disease, diabetes, hypothyroidism and oral or intravenous steroid treatment can also negatively impact a person's chances of contracting sinusitis.

In addition, risk factors such as whether or not you smoke or have been exposed to secondhand smoke can also factor significantly as to whether or not you develop sinusitis. Smoking tends to impact most health conditions, in particular respiratory conditions, so it is no real surprise that smoking can significantly increase someone's chances of developing sinusitis.

Complications

Complications can occur with every illness. It's undeniable. Sinusitis is no different, except the complications that occur can potentially be more serious as it is the respiratory system which is affected in this case. For instance, further asthma attacks may be triggered. Also, because the blood vessels in the nose are affected as a result of the swelling that occurs, the blood supply to the brain could potentially be affected and an aneurysm or other blood clot may occur.

Since sinusitis is an infection, should that infection spread into the surrounding eye sockets, vision problems and perhaps even blindness may result. Meningitis may also result; this is an inflammation of the membranes and fluid surrounding your spinal cord and brain.

In addition, conditions such as osteomyelitis – an infection of the bones of the forehead and other facial bones – can develop. Adolescent males are at particular risk for this, however. Headache, fever, and soft swelling known as Pott's puffy tumor can develop as a result of osteomyelitis. Brain infection, by far, is the most significant difficulty which can develop as a result of sinusitis, particularly frontal or sphenoid sinusitis. The infection spreads to the brain via anaerobic bacteria through the bones and blood vessels.

A decreased or even eliminated sense of smell may occur as a result of sinusitis. The reasons for this are varied, but certainly one of the chief reasons could be the fact that congestion itself has caused such a significant blockage that not much can make its way through the nasal passages, including aromas and odors. Also, with repeated sinus infections, the olfactory nerve – the nerve which helps control how we perceive smell – may become compressed or damaged.

It should also be noted that in cases where infection of the overlying skin occurs because of the sinusitis, conditions such as cellulitis can occur. Cellulitis is a bacterial infection of the dermis, or the deep layer of the skin. Generally speaking, while bacteria are usually present on the surface layer of the skin and do no harm, it is when the skin gets broken by a graze, cut or bite when infection can erupt and become serious. The infection occurs because of the streptococci or staphylococci bacteria making their way into the skin.

Conventional Medical Treatments

It's important to be mindful of the overall goal of treatment when looking at the conventional modes of treatment for sinusitis. If that is kept in mind, the path to appropriate treatment then becomes clear.

There are four chief goals to treating sinusitis:

- draining the nasal passages, which become plugged;

- reducing inflammation;

- reducing the number of flare ups which occur,

- and, of course, eliminating the underlying cause.

This last goal may take some time to figure out, and there may be no ready answers. It therefore becomes incumbent on the medical professionals to alleviate the discomfort the patient is suffering. As a result, there are a variety of current conventional treatments.

Saline nasal spray will be suggested as the first line of defense in the sinusitis battle. Because of the overabundance of mucus likely present, it is important to keep the nasal passages rinsed where possible to prevent further infection and other complications. The spray is easily available in most stores, keeps things moist when the passages may be drying out as a result of the mucus, and helps clean out the nasal passages when they appear to be most plugged.

Nasal corticosteroids help eliminate and prevent inflammation. Many of these can be available over the counter, but for the most part, you have to go to a doctor to get a prescription. Examples include, but are not limited to:

- Fluticasone (Flonase);

- Budesonide (Rhinocort Aqua);

- Triamcinolone (Nasocort AQ);

- Mometasone (Nasonex);

- Beclomethasone (Beconase AQ)

Oral and injectable steroids are particularly effective when the patient is dealing with nasal polyps. Generally speaking, the patient with nasal polyps may experience extreme inflammation, which can be quite painful. Prednisone and methylprednisolone may be prescribed as a way to relieve pain and inflammation. Oral steroids are serious medications, however, with equally serious side effects; generally speaking, these are used to alleviate serious asthma conditions.

Decongestants are, for the most part, available in over-the-counter (OTC) dosings, and include such examples as Sudafed and Actifed. Generally speaking, they are only prescribed for a few days; taking these medications for any longer than that can cause a condition called *rebound congestion*. Rebound congestion is generally more severe and can create greater problems for patients dealing with sinusitis. In essence, rebound congestion is simply congestion which has become worse with the ongoing use of traditional over-the-counter medications. Rather than being a true "rebound", what happens is that the person has become unwittingly addicted to the spray. What happens is that in seeking relief from the symptoms of sinusitis or congestion, the person using the nasal spray may increase the dosing slightly or continue to use it in the hopes that the spray will ultimately improve symptoms. It is suspected that the extended use of these medications can cause the nasal passages to constrict and swell. Over the counter pain relievers may also be recommended, such as aspirin or ibuprofen. However, due to the risk of Reye's Syndrome, aspirin should never be given to anyone under 18.

Antibiotics might be required to clear up a case of sinusitis if it is brought about as a result of a bacterial infection. Usually, there is a different underlying cause for sinusitis than a bacterial infection, so antibiotics may not be useful. If it is as a result of a bacterial infection, amoxicillin or doxycycline might be prescribed to clear up the infection. It is important, of course, to take the entire course of medication.

Immunotherapy may be used in cases where allergies are contributing to the sinusitis. If allergies are a contributing factor, allergy shots may be prescribed to help reduce the body's reaction to specific allergens.

Cases which are resistant to treatment may require surgical intervention via an endoscopic surgical procedure. A thin tube with an attached light would be gently inserted into your nasal and sinus passages to explore the surrounding tissues. Tissue may be removed, a polyp may be shaved away, or even the sinus opening itself may be enlarged in order to improve drainage.

18

Chapter 2: Sinusitis Relief with Diet

Food Allergy and Diet

To understand sinusitis, it is important to look at the underlying causes of it. One significant cause of sinusitis can be food allergies, especially as the incidents of food allergies are on the rise. What's the difference between an allergy and sensitivity, however?

A food allergy can range in severity. An allergy is an immune system response which occurs shortly after eating a certain food. Responses can be as minor as hives or as serious as swollen airways. A food allergy can also cause a serious condition known as *anaphylaxis*, which can ultimately be fatal.

Food allergies affect six to eight per cent of the adult population. It is easy to confuse an allergy with an intolerance; they both imply some sort of issues in tolerating food. However, a food intolerance is far less serious and does not generally involve the immune system.

Food Allergy and Sinus Problems

So what can be done to control food allergies? Is it necessary to get a shot every time you have a reaction? Generally speaking, histamines are released when the body has an allergic response to something; this, in turn, causes inflammation and swelling in certain tissues of the body, and quite likely the mucous membranes would be involved.

The fact of the matter is, *biogenic amines* may be involved in the allergic response process. They are derived from a group of amino acids, and therefore from **protein-rich foods**. They affect the body in certain ways, both positive and negative, and may cause some issues, depending on the person's response. In addition to being amino acids, they may also function as neurotransmitters. The best known neurotransmitters include dopamine, noradrenaline, serotonin, and histamine. These biogenic amines may regulate stomach functions, be involved in the inflammation produced during histamine release in allergic responses, or may cause migraines, hives or asthma responses.

Up to five per cent of adults deal with histamine intolerance or HIT. As a result, it can be a major cause of food intolerance. Histamine intolerance (HIT) can cause low blood pressure, bloating, migraines and palpitations. It may also be involved in various digestive upsets such as diarrhea or constipation. Because of the further physiological issues involved with conditions like low blood pressure or digestive upsets, further complications like low sodium levels or electrolytes may result.

Tyramine is connected with migraines, high blood pressure, depression and Parkinson's disease. This biogenic amine can be particularly dangerous for those taking MAOI anti-depressants as its breakdown can be blocked, and this, in turn, can cause dangerously high blood pressure. Given sinusitis can, at the very least, compress blood vessels, this can complicate matters greatly.

Phenylethylamine can contribute to migraines, depression, attention deficit hyperactivity disorder and schizophrenia. When considering that sinusitis can cause throbbing headaches and such things, it's easy to see that these biogenic amines can create a great deal of difficulty when it comes to coping with sinusitis as well.

Food Intolerance and Sinus Problems

Any food can trigger an allergic response. Any food which can cause the immune system to respond can cause an allergic reaction. Food intolerances, to an extent, can create inflammation, which can, in turn, lead to sinusitis. Proper blood testing needs to be done in order to eliminate anything which can trigger the sinusitis, if the underlying cause is food-related. Unfortunately, it may take some time before the connection is made between a physiological response to food and to a sinusitis symptom.

Ingredients in Food to Avoid

Cheese, chocolate, and citrus fruit has often been labeled as the "3 Cs" of foods to avoid for those with food sensitivities. In particular, people with food allergies should avoid aged cheeses, as aged cheeses are higher in amines, which can, as mentioned, trigger allergic responses. Fish and meat can also cause significant histamine responses for those struggling with sinusitis. If the meat is grilled, people may also have an allergic response, but in reality, what has caused the reaction is the amines as opposed to the meat or fish itself.

Soybean, miso, and fermented bean curd are very high in tyrosine, which ultimately metabolises into the biogenic amine tyramine. Tyramine, as described above, can contribute to significant allergic reactions, among them the inflamed nasal passages which can be a symptom of sinusitis. Fish sauce can also contribute to allergic responses, and as a result, their consumption should be limited.

Certain wines - particularly red wines - can cause a significant allergic response. People who have a reaction to red wines may flush greatly or they may also break into hives. In fact, alcohol in general can cause a problem; beer and vermouth have also been known to cause difficulties in people. In addition, alcohol is a well-known diuretic; this means, of course, that it dehydrates the drinker. What this can result in is hardened mucus in the nasal passages, which does not allow for the person to be able to effectively clear their sinuses.

Coffee and other highly caffeinated beverages should also be avoided. Coffee is a well-known cause of heartburn, which can also contribute to acid reflux. In addition, like alcohol, coffee is also a diuretic. Coffee can cause the drinker to urinate more frequently and therefore can pull the moisture out of the person's system, which also means that hardened mucus in nasal passages and sinuses can result.

Fermented foods can also cause people who suffer from sinusitis a great deal of discomfort. This reason why fermented foods can cause a problem is because during the fermentation process, the amino acid histidine gets transformed into histamine, which is present in large quantities during the fermentation process. Foods such as aged cheeses, alcohol, eggs, strawberries and tomatoes, to name but a few, not only find their histamine counts on the rise as a result of the fermentation process, but are initially high in histamines. This means people who have histamine sensitivity need to be very aware of what they are eating and what foods or drinks cause allergic responses in order to avoid further sinus attacks.

Ingredients in food like hot sauce and horseradish seem to be the immediate go-to spices in order to promote sinus drainage. The smell of the food alone, sometimes, can thin the mucus and break it up, and instantly, you may seem a bit like a running tap. However, there is a catch: spicy foods can also trigger acid reflux, which can be a contributing factor to causing a sinusitis attack. It is almost a catch-22; the spicy foods are causing your nose – and every other mucous membrane in your head – to drain almost instantly, but you are opening yourself up to another sinus attack because of the acid reflux which may accompany the consumption of the spicy food.

The reason why acid reflux can be such a significant contributing factor to sinusitis attacks is because there is no clear-cut division between the nose and the esophagus. There is only a smooth transition, and because of this, if stomach acid climbs back into the esophagus after the consumption of spicy foods or late-night meals, sinusitis can occur.

The amount of amines in food can vary extensively, so if it is suspected that food allergies are the root cause of the sinusitis, testing should be done as soon as possible. It is also possible that things like overheating food, such as on a grill, may also increase the number of amines in food so depending on the type of food being grilled and the amount of pre-existing biogenic amines in the food, there may be a greater risk for allergic response - especially, of course, those responses which may mimic sinusitis.

In the acute stages of sinusitis, it is important for the patient to drink a lot of fresh fruit and vegetable juices diluted with water in order to beat back the fever. After the fever dies, the patient can adopt a low-calorie, balanced diet with many raw fruits and vegetables, as well as raw fruits and vegetable juices. Once the patient has recovered, he or she may gradually switch over to a well-balanced diet with an emphasis on seeds, grains, nuts, vegetables and fruit. Short juice fasts may also be of benefit to help control symptoms for a week at two month intervals.

Chapter 3: Sinusitis Relief with Nutritional Supplements

There are a variety of non-medicinal treatments that people can make use of in order to beat chronic sinusitis. The emphasis should be on at least ensuring you have the basics for vitamin and mineral support. The basics, when it comes to vitamin supplements, include Vitamins A, C and E, as well as integrating the minerals Zinc and Selenium. Even healthy people should make use of these supplements in order to improve overall health.

These vitamins and minerals belong to a special class called antioxidants, and they are designed to help cells ward off damage from free radicals, which can impair the functioning of cell membranes. The unfortunate part of daily living is our bodies do not take in or manufacture enough of these antioxidants in order to successfully ward off free radicals. As a result, we end up having to take supplements.

While some supplementation of our diets is good, sometimes people subscribe to the philosophy of "one's good, many is much better". The bottom line is, overdoing it in the vitamin and mineral department can be damaging to our systems. For instance, consuming too much vitamin C, either through diet or supplements, can cause someone to have diarrhea. While unpleasant, this condition may also be necessary; sometimes it is good to clean out the gastrointestinal tract. However, diarrhea can also throw other things out of balance, such as your electrolyte levels.

Many vitamin and mineral supplements including those discussed below are available through either your local grocery store or your pharmacist. If your town is big enough, you can also find nutritional supplements in your health food store.

- **Undecylenic acid** is a fatty acid found in the skin's sebaceous secretions. This particular fatty acid has been found to be excellent in curing fungal infections, particularly allergic fungal sinusitis. In fact, the zinc salt in undecylenic acid was used for years in antifungal pharmaceutical preparations until stronger antifungals were used. It has been used in both topical and oral antifungal preparations for years. While there has been no current large-scale clinical studies done about its efficacy, its effective use in defeating fungal infections in the past has been indisputable.

- **Bromelain** has also been used as a symptom reliever for sinusitis. It has been used as both an anti-inflammatory and a mucolytic. In fact, a 2005 German study showed that children had significantly speedier symptom recovery times while taking doses of bromelain than the control group. This confirms findings from the 1960s which stated that bromelain was effective in fighting sinusitis symptoms. It thins mucous when taken and that, of course, is key in alleviating the pain and inflammation associated with sinusitis.

- **Urtica dioica** – more commonly known as stinging nettle – may also be recommended as a method of reducing the pain and inflammation associated with sinusitis. In fact, in cases of allergic rhinitis, stinging nettle was shown to be quite effective in alleviating symptoms. The symptoms of allergic rhinitis can be quite close to those of sinusitis, and as such, can be considered as a means of treatment. Freeze-dried stinging nettle, generally administered in capsule form, can be quite useful in reducing symptoms for the simple fact that for whatever reason, it appears to alleviate the inflammation and mucous production associated with sinusitis.

- **Essential fatty acids** such as Omega-3's are also important to take, both for healthy people and for those struggling with sinusitis. The body needs to keep moist and lubricated; without it, we become very stiff, and our joints and membranes become equally tight and immovable. Taking in these fatty acids allows waste products and toxins to be eliminated from your system far more efficiently. Fatty acids also help to keep mucous membranes clear and running efficiently – something which contributes greatly to the alleviation of sinusitis symptoms.

- **Quercetin** can also be used as a method of relief from sinusitis. It is a bioflavonoid which has been proven to help reduce inflammation and boost the immune system, and is found in the skin of apples and red onions. It reduces the production of mucous by blocking the production of histamine, which has been proven to cause the swelling and mucous production associated with sinusitis and many allergic reactions.

- **N-acetyl cysteine** is an antioxidant which is an altered form of the amino acid cysteine. Its use has generally been prescribed to ease the extreme congestion found in cystic fibrosis cases, and therefore is useful in eliminating the sinus congestion which occurs in sinusitis cases.

Chronic sinusitis can also be an indication of immune system compromise. As a result, care should be taken to boost the immune system against further attacks by viruses and disease. As mentioned above, taking a supplement which contains vitamin C, vitamin E, carotene complex (which helps boost the health of mucous membranes), zinc and selenium can go a long way in promoting immune system health and therefore help in the fight against sinusitis.

Olive leaf extract and garlic have also been shown to help kill candida, or yeast. Yeast has often been theorized to be an underlying cause of sinusitis, so by eliminating candida, it is possible to eliminate the underlying cause of a sinusitis and therefore lead the patient on the road to recovery.

Chapter 4: Sinusitis Relief with Herbal Remedies

Homeopathy is a natural approach to health and healing which allows people who follow that philosophy to take very small doses of vitamins or minerals from the plant or animal kingdom to become healthy. As such, it can also be used as a relatively side-effect free approach to alleviating sinusitis symptoms.

This treatment philosophy is based on the approach that symptoms are the body's defense to infection or stress. It is also the symptoms that are displayed that help guide a homeopath's approach in determining the most effective treatment options. It is therefore important that the person suffering from sinusitis be able to pinpoint their symptoms and accurately describe them so that proper treatment may be suggested.

Homeopathic treatment can be used as a method for alleviating the symptoms of acute sinusitis, but it is important to keep in mind that the more serious, chronic sinusitis symptoms should still be treated by a medical professional. There are several herbal approaches, and while on their own they might be poisonous, they are generally sold in such high dilutions that their purposes are generally medicinal in value.

- **Echinacea** (purple coneflower) and **goldenseal** can be useful in boosting the immune system in order to ward off future infections. In addition, it is believed that goldenseal has a unique ability to clear mucus out of congested nasal passages, thereby reducing the inflammation and pain of sinusitis. It should be noted that Echinacea does carry with it some side effects. Nausea and heartburn can be common with prolonged use of Echinacea, which of course can exacerbate symptoms of sinusitis. Allergic responses may also develop, including runny nose, hay fever and the like. It can be taken in capsule form, but can also be used in a nasal rinse in order to relieve congestion. It is recommended that people only take Echinacea for no longer than two weeks without talking to their doctor, as it is possible some other ailment may be at play.

- **Teas made from ginger, elderflower, chamomile, ground ivy or peppermint** can also be very useful in terms of their properties in relieving pain and congestion.

- **Belladonna** (deadly nightshade) can be used by people experiencing over-full sinuses. Its use is generally recommended during the first stage of a sinus infection, as it can be helpful in alleviating headaches associated with sinuses which are plugged. Patients may also have the sense of the pain coming and going. People may feel aggravated at the slightest movement, which includes being jarred, nudged or other unexpected movements. There might also be a sense of improved symptoms if the patients try to maintain a semi-erect posture.

- **Mercurius** can be used for those patients who feel their heads are being squeezed in a vise. The pain may extend through to the teeth, and the patient may have difficulties in regulating their temperature, often wavering from hot to cold and sweaty to chilled. Symptoms may worsen with open air, and with eating or drinking.

- **Potassium bichromate** may be recommended as a way of alleviating thick, stringy nasal discharge and pain so intense that it feels as though the scalp hurts every time the hair is brushed. There is also pain that may extend to the bones because of the sinusitis. With these symptoms, the patient may feel better lying down, being warm, drinking warm drinks and overeating.

- **Pulsatilla** (windflower) may be helpful when the sinusitis has developed after being overheated, and symptoms may be worse when the patient is lying down. Patients requiring pulsatilla treatment may find that their symptoms improve when they wrap their heads tightly with a bandage or when lying down in a cool room. Their pain may shift from one area of the head to another, and symptoms may improve when cold compresses are applied.

- **Silicea** may be considered for those whose congestion seems chronic. Head pain seems to be worse on the right side, particularly in the right eye, and may worsen with cold, movement, light and mental concentration, such as that which occurs when studying.

- **Grape seed extract** can also be taken in order to help reduce inflammation of the nasal passages. It is the antioxidant properties in the grape seed extract which can work wonders in reducing inflammation in and around the nasal passages and sinus cavities. Up to 50 milligrams three times daily should be consumed in order to see relatively immediate relief from the swelling and inflammation. Other herbs that can be used include eyebright, marshmallow and goldenrod.

While knowing which is the appropriate herb to take given the appropriate symptom is important, it is also critical to discuss treatment options and decisions with a licensed naturopath or homeopath. To do otherwise would be irresponsible and potentially dangerous.

Chapter 5: Sinusitis Relief with Home Remedies

Neti Pot

Perhaps the most commonly-used home remedy to date is the **Neti Pot**. In essence, all a Neti Pot is is a nasal irrigation device designed for keeping nasal passages clean and clear. It comes from the Ayurvedic or yoga medical traditions, and is generally ceramic, though there are plastic versions of the pot available for distribution. It looks like a cross between a teapot and Aladdin's lamp. Neti Pots have been around for several years, but have actually increased in popularity as a result of their appearance on Oprah.

Generally speaking, many people are quite nervous about using a Neti Pot at first, as it requires you to pour liquid – usually a saline solution of some sort – through one nostril and let it pour freely out the other. There may be some concerns about choking on the fluid because of how you are expected to use it. The recommendation is to go see a doctor or ear, nose and throat specialist in order to get appropriate advice in using the Neti Pot.

The idea behind the Neti Pot is that it clears the *cilia* – tiny structures that line the nasal passages and sinus cavities – which wave back and forth to move mucus either to the back of the throat to be swallowed or up to the nose to be blown out. Saline solution has been shown to help improve the speed and coordination of the cilia.

To use the Neti Pot, one would mix 16 ounces of lukewarm water with one ounce of salt. Distilled, sterile or boiled water that has, of course, cooled is generally recommended; this removes any impurities which may cause some issues during the use of the Neti Pot. Then, the user's head should be tilted over a sink at a 45 degree angle and the solution should be slowly poured into one nostril.

If the angle is right, the solution should flow relatively easily out the other nostril. It is possible that some of the solution may pour into the throat during this process. If that's the case, it should just be spat out into the sink. The idea is to take your time and go slow in order to avoid the saline rinse from sliding inadvertently into the throat.

The Neti Pot has also generally been found to be quite safe in its application. In fact, only about 10 percent of users have experienced mild difficulties, ranging from nasal irritation to nosebleeds. These difficulties, however, may be remedied by regulating the frequency of use, adjusting the amounts of salt in the solution and changing the temperature of the water.

If someone is suffering from daily sinus symptoms, relief has been found from using nasal irrigation daily. Once symptoms have been alleviated, however, it is generally recommended to continue using the Neti Pot or other nasal irrigation system three times a week.

Clean the Air

Because the sinuses are designed to be a natural air filtration system, sinusitis patients may find some relief from using an air/HEPA filter combination. By using this sort of filtration system, potential allergens and pollutants, such as dust and animal dander, can be further eliminated and not have as much of an impact on an already-compromised immune system.

HEPA stands for "High Efficiency Particulate Air", and a HEPA filter can trap a very large amount of small particles which would otherwise be re-circulated into the air using traditional vacuum cleaners. This type of filtration system therefore reduces the amount of allergens that get spewed back into the air more effectively than a traditional air filter.

Using a HEPA filter can therefore make the air cleaner for the residents of your home. Using an allergen-proof pillow case and mattress may also help further cut back on the challenges to a sinusitis sufferer's immune system. In addition, using an allergen-proof vacuum filter that won't create further dust and dirt can also help greatly.

Steam

By far, one of the most common home treatments for sinusitis is the application of steam. Steam allows the mucus in the nasal passages and sinus cavities to thin somewhat, offering quick and noticeable relief from symptoms. In addition, it has been noted that particularly hot steam can provide some germ-killing properties, though some medical specialists may argue that the steam landing on surfaces can cause a build-up of moisture and therefore encourage the development of mold.

If a couple of drops of eucalyptus oil are also added, this can help combat the infection. Rest, sleep and lots of fresh air can be critical components in the battle against sinus trouble.

Avoid Perfumes and Scented Hair Oils

Perfumes and scented hair oils should be avoided, as these can trigger allergic responses, which can worsen symptoms. The chemical composition of these perfumes and scented hair oils, which are generally manufactured and not of natural composition, can trigger allergic responses, causing inflammation of the nasal passages and potentially the sinus cavities. Instead, natural essential oil fragrances with diffusers should be used. The essential oils found in nature can be gentler on the system than those manufactured in a factory and as such, are kinder to those suffering from sinusitis.

Compresses

It should also be noted that warm and cool compresses can also be used to help bring relief. The warm compresses can be used to ease tense muscles and the cool can be used to help reduce swelling, or at the very least, the sensation of it. That, in and of itself, can be of great comfort to the person dealing with sinusitis, as frequently the pain and discomfort they experience seems never to abate.

A ginger compress can also be prepared in order to give optimum sinus pain relief. A quarter cup of actual ginger root should be grated and put into a pint of boiling water. The results should then be strained and the water then used to soak a cloth to be used as a compress. This should help with the nasal drainage, and with luck, eliminate the sinus issues.

Horseradish

Horseradish can also be used as a method of clearing sinuses during sinusitis. One teaspoon of horseradish should be mixed with a half teaspoon of olive oil and one teaspoon of lemon juice. The mixture can then be either consumed directly or mixed with rice or potatoes if a burning sensation is experienced while consuming it.

The bottom line is, symptom treatment and relief depends on the underlying causes.

46

Chapter 6: Sinusitis Relief with Alternative Therapies

Acupuncture

Acupuncture, as a sinusitis-relief therapy, has often been considered as a key method in fighting the congestion and inflammation associated with this extremely-uncomfortable condition. Western medicine doesn't usually ascribe to the theories involved with acupuncture as a sinusitis treatment, and those who are suffering with the infection may begin looking for alternative treatment measures in order to gain more permanent relief without the potential side effects associated with more traditional-based medical therapies.

Under traditional Chinese medical beliefs, there are several potential symptoms at play in both chronic and acute sinusitis:

- Lung/spleen dampness

- Lung heat

- Lung/spleen damp heat

- Large intestine channel disturbance

- Qi (Chi) stagnation

- Lung disturbance

Lung/Spleen dampness means there could be congestion in the lungs and/or spleen. It's possible that the person struggling with sinusitis could live in a damp environment and spend a lot of time in the rain. Tangible signs of dampness may include phlegm, edema (swelling) and oozing from open sores. There may also be an overall sense of heaviness; since things that are damp have a tendency to sink, the dampness in the body may "sink" towards the lower organs.

Lung heat means there could be an excess of yellow mucous in the lungs, which means that manipulation of the acupuncture points associated with the affected organ can help alleviate symptoms of sinusitis. Herbs can also be used in conjunction with the acupuncture in order to clear the excess heat.

Lung/Spleen damp heat means the person experiencing this may experience symptoms of thirst without having any real desire to drink, have the symptoms of heaviness associated with lung/spleen dampness, nausea and headaches.

Large intestine channel disturbance indicates that the person may be experiencing dry mouth, shivering, cold, dizziness, constipation and bowels that appear to rumble.

Qi (Chi) stagnation means the patient may experience headache or dizziness, a tight abdomen or bloating.

To treat sinusitis via acupuncture, several different acupuncture points may be used, including those in the ears or along the side of the nose. White flower oil may also be applied under the nose in order to help encourage the flow of energy among the various affected organs and restore good health.

Acupuncture is not, however, to be undertaken by a layperson. There are people who are specifically licensed and trained to administer acupuncture as a holistic means of recovery from illness and disease. There is a very specific means of inserting the specialized needles under the skin in order to promote positive health and recovery from illness. It should not be done by anyone from home; it is a method of practicing Eastern medicine which is only to be done under controlled, sanitized circumstances and conditions.

Acupressure

Acupressure and acupuncture should not be confused. Where acupuncture must be done by a trained and licensed acupuncturist and involves a variety of long, thin needles, acupressure is something which can be done by yourself wherever you are.

Acupressure is based on the philosophy that there are certain areas on the sinuses which are particularly sensitive to bioelectric impulses and that these areas can be manipulated gently in order to restore good health. Stimulation of these points by using either heat or pressure can trigger the neurochemical endorphin to relieve pain and tension. Of course, endorphins are naturally released while doing various physical activities and help the person engaging in these activities feel good. Endorphins are a natural pain killer.

Stimulating these sinus pressure points do not necessarily hit the root of the sinus issue –

such as infections or allergens – but they can offer relief from the sinusitis itself by helping encourage the free flow of the cilia, the tiny hairs in the nose which help promote the flow of mucus out of the nose. It is important to manipulate these sinus pressure points properly and as frequently as necessary in order to keep the nasal passages clear and free-flowing as possible. By doing so, the continued health of nasal passages and sinus cavities is promoted.

The areas around the nose, in particular the base of the nose where the nostrils flare out, should be pressed with a fair degree of pressure, with special attention being paid to the cheeks as well. Applying a fair bit of pressure can help with pain relief and help aid mucous drainage, which is a significant problem with sinusitis.

Reflexology

Reflexology is, in a nutshell, using pressure points, generally on the patient's foot, in order to achieve some sort of medical benefit elsewhere in the body. One of the most common places to practice reflexology is in the foot.

There are a series of sinus reflex points in the foot, both in the toes and just underneath them. When reflexology is practiced, the patient may feel a great deal of pain, as the sinus pressure points may feel like a pinhead under the thumb. This can send a great deal of pain through the patient, so a good reflexologist needs to be aware of the amount of pressure he or she is using.

It should be noted that while reflexology can provide almost immediate relief from the pain and discomfort, it is not a cure all for sinusitis itself. What it does do, however, is provide the person suffering from sinusitis increased blood circulation to the nose and sinus area. This, in turn, provides the sufferer almost immediate relief from the congestion which blocks their nose and sinuses and eases the pain they may be experiencing.

Before beginning any reflexology to clear sinuses, the patient should drink a glass of water, if possible. This will help promote circulation to key areas, in this case, the nose and sinuses.

The tips of all toes on the right foot, and then the tips of all fingers on the same side, should be squeezed gently for five seconds each. Depending on how plugged the sinuses are, it is possible that this procedure could be very painful for the patient going through treatment. The meridian points on the toes – generally somewhere just under the nail or at the front of the toe – should be gently stimulated in a circular and clockwise motion, and then a counter-clockwise motion, for ten seconds each.

The sinus points on all toes should gently be worked on, followed by gentle massage of the sinus ridge underneath the toes, for roughly two minutes per foot. This procedure should be repeated several times over the course of a visit. If it's been done effectively, the sinuses should begin to drain with little effort.

There are also fifteen sinus pressure points on the face which can be stimulated in order to promote drainage, and therefore relief, for those dealing with sinusitis. Approximately one minute per pressure point should be spent in order to help alleviate symptoms, which means that even as a do-it-yourself remedy, facial reflexology should take no more than fifteen minutes.

In addition, applying pressure to the adrenal reflex areas of the hand with a golf ball can help alleviate sinus issues. While reflexology sessions can be excellent at relieving symptoms, using a golf ball and sufficient pressure on the hands has been proven to help alleviate sniffles, sinusitis and sinus headaches.

Massage

Generally speaking, Western massage techniques don't appear to be very effective in the elimination of sinusitis symptoms. It appears that techniques such as Shiatsu, which make use of the body's pressure points in order to eliminate tension and balance the body's energy, are more effective in combating symptoms of sinusitis.

Issues such as sinusitis are seen as a block to the body's energy flow, and the long strokes of massage techniques such as Shiatsu are used in releasing that blockage. Because of the multiple pressure points on the face, the massage therapist will use massage techniques on the patient's face in order to clear that blocked energy.

Sinus massage can go a long way in promoting movement of mucus out of the nasal passages and sinus cavities. Beginning from the midline, massage should be conducted in small lateral circles over the forehead, towards the temples, the base and sides of the nose to the cheeks and ears. This helps to promote efficient drainage of the sinuses and reduce pain.

Cranial sacral therapy – another form of massage – can move unmoving cerebrospinal fluid within the bones of the skull. This, in turn, promotes circulation and helps ease sinus pain. This technique is particularly useful when trying to clear head, eye, ear and jaw pain during a sinus infection.

This form of therapy has been around since the 1930s, when osteopath William Garner Sutherland first suggested that since there were seams in the human skull, these areas where the seams were present could be gently manipulated in order to improve health and overall well-being. Only gentle pressure is applied to the skull; because of this and the technique's non-invasive nature, there is minimal risk to the patient. The practitioner must be able to "listen" with his or her hands to detect the cranial rhythmic impulse, which is distinct from the heart rate or regular breathing patterns. Generally speaking, there are about 10 cycles of this impulse per minute, and issues with abdominal discomfort and sinus infections can disrupt this impulse. Abnormal tension patterns can cause migraines, dizziness and sinus problems as well.

Once the therapist detects the issues with the impulse, he or she will perform the cranial sacral manipulation, and patients may feel almost immediate relief within moments of treatment. However, they may feel slightly worse for a couple of days following treatment, though rapid improvement after this immediate "settling" should occur. Therapy usually occurs once a week and shouldn't last for a long term.

Lymphatic drainage massage, when applied properly to lymph vessels in the neck and head, can help thin out mucus and therefore can help with drainage as well as reduce congestion and sinus pressure. Lymphatic drainage massage concentrates on the lymph nodes under the jaw line.

During the massage, the muscles are prewarmed and the lymph nodes are stimulated to open and enhance circulatory flow. Lymphatic drainage massage can also loosen the congestive material in the sinuses, which of course can help sinusitis sufferers feel relief from their symptoms. It then allows the lymph or healing system to do what it was trained to do – eliminate toxins in the body.

It is important, however, to note that a massage therapist, even when properly trained, will have no effective way to determine whether or not the congestion is non-infectious in nature, and so, appropriate precautions should be taken to ensure that any potential infection does not spread from patient to therapist.

Ayurvedic Medicine

Ayurvedic medicine originated from India, and is a medical system which has been around for some 2,500 years. In spite of its longevity, it is only now enjoying increasing popularity throughout health care in India, but is also spreading worldwide. According to Ayurveda, symptoms and causes of sinusitis may vary according to each person's dosha – their bodies' governing principles. Regardless of the cause, it's putting the kapha in balance – the system which regulates mucous and fluids in the sinus cavities – which allows recovery from a sinus infection or sinusitis.

Light, warm meals which are easy to digest should be the foundation of a patient's recovery when dealing with sinusitis. Steamed vegetables, cooked whole grains and fruits, and non-creamy vegetable soups should be dominant in a sinusitis patient's diet. Consumption of alcohol, which can promote the stimulation of mucous membranes, should be avoided altogether. Congestion and pressure, which are the predominant symptoms of sinusitis, can be relieved with frequent sips of hot beverages, such as herbal teas.

Due to an ongoing history of sinus infections, which is key when delivering an overall diagnosis of sinusitis, a weakened immune system is likely also at play. According to Ayurvedic principles, a weak immune system and a weak digestive system go hand in hand. As a result, eating foods which are not easily digested can produce a sticky toxin called ama, which then travels to weakened areas of the body. In this case, the sinuses would be the primary target, having already been hit by multiple infections. As a result, normal functioning of the sinuses is blocked and disease can erupt.

The best way to clear the body of toxins is to boil spring water and sip it throughout the day. For really effective results during sinus attacks, steeping two slices of fresh ginger, four leaves of fresh mint, two cloves, and one teaspoon of marshmallow root can help destroy the toxic *ama*. The tea should be kept hot all day in a thermos and sipped throughout the day. In addition, cooking with digestion and immune-enhancing spices such as turmeric, ginger, cumin, coriander, fennel, and black pepper can help in recovery.

Under the Ayurvedic discipline, sinus problems are suspected to have their roots in the digestive system. In essence, when people eat, there is a pure part which is drawn off to nourish the body and then there's the refuse, which is left behind. It's thought that the digestive juices, in essence, don't do enough to break down the refuse, so what's left in the system spreads throughout the body and creates some damage.

There could be many reasons, under traditional thought, as to why the fluid tends to accumulate in the nose. There could be stress-related issues, emotional issues, or anything like that. According to Ayurvedic philosophy, these are the immediate disease-causing factors. Over time, if the accumulation of mucous and disruption of air flow continues, the entire tissues of the face can become distorted. Muscles tense, bone structure becomes compressed and nerves pinch. Tightness and pain results. This, in turn, can lead to vision loss, early greying of hair, and skin wrinkling.

Other Homeopathic Cures for Sinusitis

It's important to take good care of yourself in order to have a better chance at combating most illnesses and diseases which may come down the pipe and attack throughout the course of any given year. Maintaining a healthy immune system is important when it comes to bolstering your resources in battling germs. In addition, staying in shape, eating right and getting plenty of rest are critical in order to be effective in fighting infections and disease.

Living a clean life is also important; whether you have to wash your hands following going to the bathroom or using antibacterial sanitizer in order to keep yourself as germ-free as possible, it's important to take necessary precautions to stay healthy. That includes washing hands, not sharing utensils or glasses with anyone and generally speaking, avoiding contact with those who are dealing with an infectious illness can all contribute to not getting sick.

As always, staying hydrated is a good plan in general. Eight tall glasses of water can go a long way in staving off illnesses including sinusitis. In addition, the consumption of water goes a long way in promoting good circulation throughout all parts of the body, including the nose and sinuses.

It's also important to avoid air pollutants in general, including cigarette smoke. Cigarette smoke can be one of the greatest contributing factors to having a sinusitis attack and if you are in constant exposure to cigarette smoke, or are a smoker yourself, you are only asking for further health issues. In addition, if there is a smog advisory or the news has reported that the air quality is poor in your area, stay indoors. You'll be doing yourself a favor.

If you do have allergies, it is important to learn a variety of techniques to deal with allergens present in your environment in order to avoid future sinusitis attacks. Learning desensitization techniques can help you learn tools to avoid future sinusitis attacks. It's also important to be aware of what allergens cause difficulties for you and then avoid them.

Consuming apple cider vinegar can also go a long way to thinning mucus and clearing blocked sinus cavities. Long thought of as a method of controlling appetite, apple cider vinegar can help people lose and control weight, which has long been considered key in the battle against sinusitis.

Drinking a mix of apple cider vinegar and water prior to symptoms of sinusitis actually starting helps to alleviate those initial symptoms of sinusitis. These initial symptoms include watery eyes, a stuffy nose, and a sinus headache. In fact, consuming a blend of apple cider vinegar and water has been shown to transform mucus from a thick, green or yellow appearance to clear and thin. Thinning the mucus is the first step to beating back a sinus infection; once the mucus has been thinned, other more effective means of eliminating the infection can be pursued.

Using wild oregano oil has been thought of as a good method in beating back colds and sinus infections. Before using an essential oil such as wild oregano oil, it is important to ensure that the oil is diluted with something such as olive oil, simply because essential oils in and of themselves are far too strong and potent to be used on their own.

Wild oregano oil is also a skin irritant and therefore should be consumed with other foods or juices in order to dilute their effects. In addition, women who are pregnant should not use oregano oil, as it is an abortifacient and therefore can cause miscarriage. Diabetics shouldn't use wild oregano oil either, as it has the potential for lowering blood sugar.

Since tomatoes and garlic, as well as hot peppers, have been known for their medicinal value because they are high in vitamin C, some people have believed that a spicy tomato tea works very well in the alleviation of sinus pain from sinusitis. With a balance of tomato juice, a few cloves of garlic and as much hot sauce as can be tolerated, small wonder that people are experiencing sinuses that become clear fairly quickly.

To make an effective spicy tomato tea, take two cups of V-8 or other tomato juice, two or three cloves of garlic – more if it can be tolerated – two tablespoons of lemon juice, and as much hot sauce as can be tolerated. Ingredients should be mixed and heated in a pan or microwave. Contents should be re-warmed as needed in order to get the full benefit of the fumes.

It is the hot sauce and garlic, in particular, which will work wonders in alleviating symptoms of sinusitis. Capsaicin, one of the chief ingredients in hot sauce, has been found to be soothing to the stomach and throat, and has excellent anti-fungal and anti-bacterial properties. In fact, capsaicin has been found to be very effective in killing Candida, a fungal infection which has been found to be responsible for many physical issues we have, including allergies.

As mentioned in the Chapter 3, however, that while spicy foods can go a long way in seeming to alleviate sinusitis, it is possible that they may exacerbate symptoms of acid reflux, which can, in turn, contribute to future sinusitis attacks.

Summary

Sinus infections and, in particular, sinusitis are some of the most aggravating conditions for people to deal with. Colds are generally bad enough; unfortunately, sinusitis is like the worst cold you have ever had to the nth degree. There is no real immediate relief from the excessive sinus congestion, and it seems as though it can consume every aspect of your daily routine. You have difficulties breathing due to blocked nasal passages and sinuses, there could be a headache which comes and goes, and a great deal of sensitivity to cold, light, or pressure. Your mood can also be significantly impacted, as you don't feel well in the first place and, in the second place, there seems to be no real answers – medically, at least – as to how to relieve symptoms quickly and get some time that seems to be pain-free.

Over the years, people have tried a variety of different approaches to try and alleviate the pain of sinusitis. The most popular remedy that seems to have caught on – largely thanks to the influence of Oprah – is the Neti Pot, a smallish sort of a teapot that people can use to run a saline rinse through their sinuses. In spite of some concerns by the population which are largely unfounded about the risks of gagging while pouring the rinse through, the Neti Pot's use continues to be on the rise.

Allergens can be the biggest culprit in causing a sinus flare-up. Dust, dirt, pollen and other things can cause a sinusitis attack. Allergens can cause the mucous membranes to swell and the nose to become blocked as a result. The sinuses begin to fill with mucous, and because the nasal passages are blocked, the sinuses cannot drain effectively.

Over-the-counter decongestants and nasal sprays can be used to alleviate symptoms, but their use is limited because if the sprays are used longer than a few days, rebound congestion can occur. Rebound congestion is when nasal sprays and decongestants have been used longer or in greater dosages than is actually recommended. It is also, in essence, when addiction to the nasal spray has occurred; the person using the spray has now got a system which is used to the spray's presence, and so it may seem more spray is required. This constricts the nasal passages and can lead to swelling therein.

Sometimes, this rebound congestion can worsen the condition that initially underwent treatment. The only thing that can improve a condition like rebound congestion is stoppage of the nasal sprays for a few days. That will allow the nasal passages an opportunity to recover.

Nutritional supplements and herbs have also proven to be quite useful in the battle against sinusitis, provided that the patient is also taking care to get plenty of rest, avoid substances which can cause an allergic response – which can, in turn, worsen symptoms of sinusitis and sinus infections – and also drink plenty of water. The reason why water is critical in sinusitis recovery is because water helps lubricate the body's systems, and it also helps in boosting circulation throughout the essential areas of the body, including the nose and sinus cavities. Water can also help flush toxins out of the body, thereby allowing the build-up of mucus potentially to drain more effectively.

Eastern medical traditions have also been investigated as a method in battling sinusitis and sinus infections as well. In the Ayurvedic tradition, it is believed that a weakened immune system goes hand in hand with a weakened digestive system and as such, greater care should be taken with the sufferer's diet.

The sinusitis patient should consider lighter meals that are far easier to digest rather than ones that may contribute to further digestive and nasal upsets. The Ayurvedic medical principles state that by consuming easily digestible meals, patients will cut down on the sticky toxin *ama* which is often present when infections such as sinusitis occur. Ama is the toxin responsible for the manufacture of mucous and inflammation throughout the nasal passages and sinus cavities.

Acupuncture and acupressure can also go a long way in relieving sinusitis symptoms. Where acupressure can be done on your own, in a time frame as short as fifteen minutes, acupuncture must be done under controlled conditions with a trained acupuncturist.

Massage therapy and reflexology can also be quite useful, particularly when you think that most of the pressure points for the sinuses are either in the feet, hands or face. This form of treatment can take limited time as well.

By far, the most common and simple remedies for sinusitis are steam and saline rinses. Steam, of course, is the easiest and likely the cheapest. It is a form of treatment which can be used several times per day and can result in almost immediate relief. Unfortunately, because of the dampness which can result from its use, there may be mould residues which form on surfaces should the area where steaming is occurring is not cleaned after.

Saline rinses – whether in the form of a spray or an actual rinse administered via the use of a Neti-Pot – are generally thought to be quite safe and without side effects. However, there are some potential risks associated with using saline rinses. Firstly, the water used in the Neti-Pot may be too warm, resulting in potential injury to the soft and sensitive mucous membranes. In addition, if too much salt is used in the rinse, this can potentially have an abrasive sort of effect on the nasal passages and therefore result in nosebleeds. This of course can then cause more discomfort for the sinusitis sufferer.

It seems as though spicy foods, such as chicken wings and horseradish, can stem the pain and discomfort sinusitis and sinus infections can cause, but in reality, it is possible that they can actually make symptoms worse in the long run. This is because of a combination of factors. Firstly, there is no clear-cut division between the nose and the esophagus. Spicy foods have long been contributors to acid reflux disease, and acid reflux has been suspected as a contributing factor to sinusitis. If someone experiences an acid reflux flare, it is possible that they may also have a sinusitis attack because of the seamless path between the nose and esophagus.

Other natural remedies such as wild oregano oil have been promoted as methods of cutting mucous and preventing colds. However, it is not as simple as just consuming a few doses of oregano oil and smelling spicy for a few hours after. Oregano oil can cause a variety of issues for pregnant women and diabetics and as such, its use should be carefully considered beforehand.

Vitamin C, of course, has been widely promoted as the vitamin to consume when fighting a cold or other sinus-type infection. Fortunately, there are a variety of foods which are very high in this substance, including garlic, onions, tomatoes and oranges. In fact, there are those who swear by consuming a full clove of garlic at least once or twice a day in order to get rid of sinus troubles.

Apple cider vinegar has been thought to combat a variety of issues associated with sinus complaints. It can help control appetite, which can be useful as it has been thought that obesity is a risk factor in contracting sinusitis. In addition, apple cider vinegar has the rather unique ability to thin mucous and therefore is a great first step in the battle against sinusitis.

In short, sinusitis is a highly uncomfortable, unpleasant condition which can be caused by a variety of factors, including allergies and infections. It is important to understand the underlying causes of sinusitis before treatment options should be considered, as if conventional medical treatments are pursued, these may not be very effective. Antibiotics, in general, are ideal for bacterial infections, but do not usually target fungal infections. As such, different treatment options must also be pursued if the sinusitis is believed to be caused by a fungal infection.

It is also important to understand that treatments, whether they are natural or conventional in nature, may not necessarily treat the underlying causes of the sinusitis. Generally speaking, treatments may be more effective in dealing with the actual symptoms of the sinusitis or sinus infection rather than dealing with the actual root causes.

However, by treating the symptoms, such as thick mucus, more effective ways of tackling the sinus infection may present themselves. Eliminating or at the very least alleviating the issue of thick mucus, which blocks the sinuses and nasal passages and therefore causes the inflammation and nasal obstructions which are the hallmarks of a sinusitis diagnosis, allows for more effective treatment of the root infection.

Does conventional medical knowledge have all the answers for curing something that is surprisingly common but equally difficult to really treat effectively? No. However, eastern medical philosophies may not necessarily be effective for all sufferers of sinusitis or sinus infections either. It is important, as with any medical or health-related difficulties, to consult appropriate health care professionals, regardless of whether they are doctors, homeopaths or the like. It is also critical to realize that there is no one magic answer for curing sinusitis, but that the answers may lie in combining treatment approaches. If patients do so, they may find themselves living sinusitis-free.

Printed in Great Britain
by Amazon